40 DAYS
to
Wholeness

DESTINY IMAGE BOOKS BY BENI JOHNSON

The Happy Intercessor

The Joy of Intercession: A 40 Day Encounter
(Happy Intercessor Devotional)

Walking in the Supernatural (co-authored with Bill Johnson)

Healthy and Free

Healthy and Free Curriculum

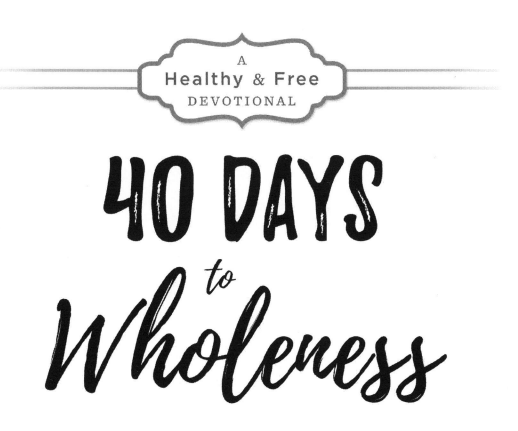

A
Healthy & Free
DEVOTIONAL

40 DAYS
to
Wholeness

BODY, SOUL & SPIRIT

BENI JOHNSON

DESTINY IMAGE® PUBLISHERS, INC.

P.O. Box 310, Shippensburg, PA 17257-0310

"Promoting Inspired Lives."

This book and all other Destiny Image and Destiny Image Fiction books are available at Christian bookstores and distributors worldwide.

Cover design by Eileen Rockwell
Interior design by Terry Clifton

For more information on foreign distributors, call 717-532-3040.

Reach us on the Internet: www.destinyimage.com.

ISBN 13 TP: 978-0-7684-1084-6
ISBN 13 eBook: 978-0-7684-1085-3

For Worldwide Distribution, Printed in the U.S.A.
1 2 3 4 5 6 7 8 / 20 19 18 17 16

CONTENTS

WEEK 1 *Day 1*   Choosing Faith over Fear 9

WEEK 1 *Day 2*   Discovering Your "Why" 13

WEEK 1 *Day 3*   You Have What It Takes. 17

WEEK 1 *Day 4*   The Weak Made Strong. 21

WEEK 1 *Day 5*   Finding Your Support Circle. 25

WEEK 2 *Day 1*   Aligning Your Thoughts with His. 31

WEEK 2 *Day 2*   Repentance: Changing Your Mind. 35

WEEK 2 *Day 3*   Letting Go of Control 39

WEEK 2 *Day 4*   The Joy of the Lord 43

WEEK 2 *Day 5*   Declare the Truth 47

WEEK 3 *Day 1*   Celebrating the Triune Connection. 53

WEEK 3 *Day 2*   The Body and Soul Connection. 57

WEEK 3 *Day 3*   Fighting Your Goliath 61

WEEK 3 *Day 4*   Where Your Emotions Reside 65

WEEK 3 *Day 5*   Respecting the Artist. 69

WEEK 4 *Day 1*   The Power of Rest 75

WEEK 4 *Day 2*   Resting in the Presence of Jesus. 79

WEEK 4 *Day 3*   Resting Is a Form of Trust. 83

WEEK 4 *Day 4*   Living Water 87

WEEK 4 *Day 5*   Water Brings Life. 91

WEEK 5 *Day 1*   Finding the Courage 97

WEEK 5 *Day 2*   Defining Success. 101

WEEK 5 *Day 3*   The Temple of God 105

WEEK 5 *Day 4*   Pressing On Toward the Goal. .109

WEEK 5 *Day 5*   Unending Grace. 113

WEEK 6 *Day 1*   One Bite of Shame. 119

WEEK 6 *Day 2*   Honoring Our Bodies with Food 123

WEEK 6 *Day 3*   Fulfillment in God. 127

WEEK 6 *Day 4*   Practicing Self-Control 131

WEEK 6 *Day 5*   The Cycle of Comparison 135

WEEK 7 *Day 1*   The Art of Loving Ourselves 141

WEEK 7 *Day 2*   Beauty in Christ. 145

WEEK 7 *Day 3*   Breaking Self-Sabotage 149

WEEK 7 *Day 4*   Accepting Your Body 153

WEEK 7 *Day 5*   Out of Hiding. 157

WEEK 8 *Day 1*   Making Time for God 163

WEEK 8 *Day 2*   The Heart of the Father 167

WEEK 8 *Day 3*   Christ Our Anchor. 171

WEEK 8 *Day 4*   Praying the Scriptures. 175

WEEK 8 *Day 5*   The Power of Worship. 179

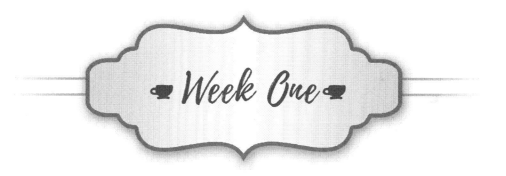

Week One

CHOOSING FAITH OVER FEAR

Jesus looked at them intently and said,
"Humanly speaking, it is impossible. But
with God everything is possible."
—MATTHEW 19:26 NLT

I still remember the day when the Lord spoke to me telling me that He wanted me to get healthy. I knew that it was the Lord, and I knew that if He wanted me to actually get healthy He would provide the way. However, the thought of it still felt overwhelming to me. Where do I begin? How long will this journey take? Will I be successful? Thoughts and questions came to my mind, and I knew that I had a choice to make. I could either allow the fear to distract me and stop me from obeying the Lord, or I could trust that God would be my source of strength.

God was faithful to me in guiding me every step of the way. I remember vividly walking into my kitchen and asking, "What do I do first, God?" My first step was to get off of sugar. So, that day, I began to educate myself and wean myself off of sugar. Little by little, I began making more positive changes into my new lifestyle.

You may be like I was, feeling overwhelmed at the road ahead of you. I encourage you to bring that fear before the Lord and lay it down. Invite Him to come alongside you on this journey, and give Him permission to instruct you along the way. He loves you and wants to be a part of every aspect of your life. It is His joy to be your guide as you move forward in learning to take care of the body that He created for you.

It is His joy to be your guide as you move forward in learning to take care of the body that He created for you.

Body

God knows what your body needs better than anybody else. Take a moment to ask God what a practical starting point for you would be. Maybe it's to begin weaning yourself off of sugar or just adding a brisk 20- to 30-minute walk into your daily routine.

Soul

The Lord wants to join you on this journey! Health was His idea in the first place! Trust that He is going to be a faithful guide and mentor.

Spirit

God, I thank You for taking me on this journey and teaching me how to be a faithful steward of my body. I ask that You quiet any fears that I may have and lead me into a place of peace and of trust. I thank You that I can trust You to fully lead me on this journey.

DISCOVERING YOUR "WHY"

Dear friend, I pray that you may enjoy good
health and that all may go well with you,
even as your soul is getting along well.
—3 JOHN 1:2 NIV

I've been blessed to be in a position where I have the opportunity to meet new people almost daily. I love being able to meet and give advice to people who have been impacted by my message of health. One of the common questions I get asked is how I am I able to stay motivated. To be honest, I am just like everybody else and there are days where I feel that I would rather sit on my couch than go to the gym. However, a tool that has helped me is discovering my "Why." Why do I want to pursue health? When God first spoke to me about becoming healthy, He told me He wanted me to be healthy because He wanted me around for the long haul. That became my "Why." Being healthy of course benefits me personally, but His statement revealed to me that there is a bigger picture at hand. My health affects the world around me. I will be unable to fulfill the call on my life if I am constantly sick and tired. Being healthy allows me to be a better wife, mother, friend, and pastor.

Motivation comes and goes for everyone. No one is exempt from that voice of temptation that wants to persuade us to eat the donuts or skip the gym. The difference between the people who keep on course and those who give up is those who stay on track see the bigger picture. Everyone is going to have a different reason for wanting to be healthy. Maybe your "Why" is to be able to live long enough to walk your daughter down the aisle or be able to take your children on adventures. Maybe your "Why" is your desire to see sickness and disease end in your family. Whatever it is, I encourage you to really sit down and find what your "Why" is.

> My health affects the world around me.
> I will be unable to fulfill the call on my
> life if I am constantly sick and tired.

Body

Take a moment to think about the ways your life would be different if you were living at your healthiest potential. What would your relationships look like? What positive impact would it have on your quality of life? Journal out what your life would look like if you really gave yourself fully to this journey of health.

Soul

Finding your "Why" is going to help keep you motivated on those days when you may be tempted to give up.

Spirit

God, I thank You that You see the bigger picture. I ask that You allow me to see this journey of health through Your eyes. Give me the grace and strength to stay the course as I venture into this lifestyle of stewarding my body and myself.

YOU HAVE WHAT IT TAKES

So do not fear, for I am with you; do not be dismayed,
for I am your God. I will strengthen you and help
you; I will uphold you with my righteous right hand.
—ISAIAH 41:10 NIV

Our society is constantly sending us messages, whether through television advertisements or in the magazine aisle of the grocery store, that we are not good enough. There is always something to fix, another pound to lose, or another way to get sculpted abs in two weeks or less. It's nearly impossible to make it through a day without something or someone sending us the message that our life could be so much better "if only."

Shame can sneak its ugly head in and begin to make us feel like we are failures. Some people try to use shame to motivate themselves to try to be better, but in the end we will never be motivated to change something we don't love.

A key to lasting change is learning to love yourself just as you are. Your body may not be at your desired weight, but it is still your body and it deserves to be loved and cared for as it is. For many of us, loving ourselves is a foreign concept because we have been so wired to want to change. However, loving ourselves is a biblical principle that Jesus spoke on. In Matthew 22, Jesus instructs the crowd to "'Love the Lord your God with all your heart, all your soul, and all your mind.' This is the first and greatest commandment. A second is equally important: 'Love your neighbor as yourself'" (Matthew 22:37–39, NLT).

Matthew 22 implies that in order to truly love each other we must be able to truly love ourselves. Part of loving ourselves means letting go of what we think we should be and embracing what and where we are. Only then will we be able to really see ourselves the way God sees us, and once we see ourselves in the light of God, we can't help but want to motivate ourselves out of a desire to love God and ourselves better.

> Part of loving ourselves means letting go of what we think we should be and embracing what and where we are.

Body

I encourage you to get before the Lord and ask Him to reveal to you how He sees you. Journal what His response is and keep it in a place that you can easily have access to in those moments when self-hate and shame try to creep in.

Soul

Lasting change can only come from a place of love. Trying to change something we hate is just a tireless race that has no end in sight. Loving ourselves will not only help us become more in tune with ourselves, but also more in tune with the Lord and others.

Spirit

God, I thank You that You have great joy in who I am. I thank You that You created me to be loved and accepted, not only by others but also by myself. I ask that You reveal to me how You see me. Show me the joys that I bring to Your heart, and please help keep my mind in alignment with those thoughts.

THE WEAK MADE STRONG

Let the weak say, "I am strong."
—JOEL 3:10 KJV

One of the greatest lies many of us have to face is the lie that we are not good enough. Who can blame us? We live in a culture where everything is constantly changing—from technology to fashion to even the ideal body type. It's impossible to keep up! In a world like we have today, the lies that we will never measure up, never be good enough, or never have what it takes can easily take root in our mind if we are not careful to guard our hearts.

The good news is that we were never created to be "good enough." Second Corinthians says, "'My grace is sufficient for you, for my power is made perfect in weakness.' Therefore I will boast all the more gladly about my weaknesses, so that Christ's power may rest on me" (2 Cor. 12:9 NIV). We were created to be dependent on God! It is His joy to meet us in our place of weakness and provide the strength and grace that we need to be able to persevere.

We all have different areas of weakness that, if given the power, can bring us shame. However, once we open ourselves up to partnering with God, those areas of weakness can become our greatest source of strength!

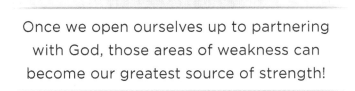

Once we open ourselves up to partnering with God, those areas of weakness can become our greatest source of strength!

Body

What are the areas of your life that you feel aren't "good enough"? Take out a journal and write those areas out. When you are done, go back through and write out the truth about those areas! Allow God to show you His perspective on what you feel are your weaknesses.

Soul

You weren't created to "be it all." One of the beautiful parts of the human experience is allowing God to move in those areas where we feel we aren't good enough. His strength becomes our strength when we partner with Him.

Spirit

God, I thank You that You already see my areas of lack. I thank You that those areas don't surprise or scare You! I invite You to come and move in my life. I surrender my desire to try to balance it all and ask that You partner with me. I ask for Your strength to become my strength.

FINDING YOUR SUPPORT CIRCLE

Two are better than one, because they have
a good return for their labor: if either of them
falls down, one can help the other up.
—ECCLESIASTES 4:9-10 NIV

One of my greatest joys in life are my girlfriends. There is nothing like having a group of girls who know everything about you and celebrate you just as you are. I have a small group of girlfriends, and we keep in contact through an ongoing group text. It allows us to laugh, process, and offer encouragement into each other's lives. In a way, these girls are my support circle.

Let us think of ways to motivate one another to acts of love and good works. And let us not neglect our meeting together, as some people do, but encourage one another, especially now that the day of his return is drawing near (Hebrews 10:24-25 NLT).

We were created to have healthy community that builds us up and helps carry us in our times of weakness. As in any journey, having a support system is essential for our success. It has been said, "If you want to go fast, go alone. If you want to go far, go together."

I encourage you to find your "people" who can act as your support circle. These people will be the ones who will celebrate your victories and help remind you of your strength when you want to give up. Allow yourself to be vulnerable in the process and allow them to really see *you*. I promise, having a group of people who support you will make all the difference as you pursue this journey to health.

> "If you want to go fast, go alone. If you want to go far, go together."

Body

Who are your cheerleaders in life? I encourage you to bring them into this journey along with you. Be open about your goals, your fears, and what you need from them! If you don't have any close friends, ask God to highlight some people to whom you can go and invite them on this journey.

Soul

We were not created to be independent of community. Having close community will only bring us closer to our goals and closer to the Father.

Spirit

God, I thank You that You have placed people in my life who can help cheer me on. I thank You that I do not have to go this journey alone and that I can be vulnerable in this process. Please give me the grace to be vulnerable and to allow myself to be seen.

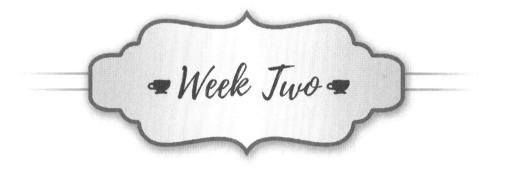

Week Two

ALIGNING YOUR THOUGHTS WITH HIS

Jesus replied: "Love the Lord your God with all your
heart and with all your soul and with all your mind."
—MATTHEW 22:37 NIV

Before we begin this week, I want to make clear the difference between the soul and the spirit. A great definition that I found is this: the soul is "the essential life of man 'looking earthward' and the 'spirit' is the same principle of life breathed (like wind) into man from God, that can look towards and experience God."[1] When I refer to the "soul," I am referring to our mind.

Our mind is one of the most powerful tools that God has given us. Dr. Caroline Leaf states that, "The mind has the power of intellect, emotions and free will, and, if enabled by the spirit and empowered by the Holy Spirit, can make good choices that can positively change the body, which includes the brain."[2] With that said, we should be very careful to be aligning our thoughts with God's truths.

In John 5:19 Jesus states, "Very truly I tell you, the Son can do nothing by himself; he can do only what he sees his Father doing, because whatever the Father does the Son also does" (NIV). This statement is powerful because it shows that Jesus was intentional about aligning His mind and soul with the Father's. The thoughts that we allow to take root inside of us can either bring us closer to the Father and align us with our destiny or draw us away making us feel disconnected.

Aligning our minds with God's not only helps us feel more connected to Him, but it is also an act of worship as we honor what the Father honors. Bill Johnson says, "I cannot afford to have a thought in my head about me that is not in His." How true this is.

> The thoughts that we allow to take root inside of us can either bring us closer to the Father and align us with our destiny or draw us away, making us feel disconnected.

Body

Take a moment to think through the last 24 hours. Think about where you went, what you did, and who you interacted with. What thoughts were you having in those moments? Take out a journal and write out the thoughts that came to your mind. If they weren't thoughts that align with what God says about you, I want you to ask God to reveal the truth to you and next to the negative thoughts write the truth that God shows you.

Soul

Our souls play an important part in having a healthy lifestyle. If we don't learn to love ourselves and align our mind with the Lord's, we will only be walking an uphill battle.

Spirit

Father, I thank You for the mind that You have given me. I give You permission to make me aware of the thoughts and mindsets that I carry that do not bring You honor. Please help lead me on this journey as I learn to align my mind, will, and emotions with You.

Notes

1. Mike, "Trichotomous vs Dichotomous Views of Man," Christianity Stack Exchange, August 7, 2012, http://christianity.stackexchange.com/questions/8847/trichotomous-vs-dichotomous-views-of-man/8887#8887.
2. Caroline Leaf, "The Mind Changes the Brain," Drleaf.com, June 1, 2015, http://drleaf.com/blog/the-mind-changes-the-brain.

REPENTANCE: CHANGING YOUR MIND

Produce fruit in keeping with repentance.
—MATTHEW 3:8 NIV

We've all been there before. We are desperate to make a change. We see its importance and we may even know the exact steps to take to get us there, but something keeps holding us back—the past. Maybe it's memories of failed attempts you've made in the past or a hurtful comment someone once made to you. Whatever it is, it is time to let it go.

We are all familiar with the apostle Paul. He still stands as one of the influential evangelists and ministers of Christ. His revelations about God still bring comfort to people today. Can you imagine having that much influence, to the point where people are still talking about you over 2,000 years after your life? He lived a life of such excellence that it's easy to forget that before his life of travels, missionary work, and promoting of the gospel Paul was once Saul.

Saul was known for his violence against Christians and his complete disregard toward Christ. However, that didn't stop God from handpicking him and using what was once his greatest weakness to become his greatest strength. Even after Saul's encounter with the Lord, he had a choice to make. Would he deny Jesus and choose to stay an angry and bitter Pharisee or would he accept this invitation to a transformed life? Thankfully, he choose the latter and the world is still reaping the benefits of his choice.

The word *repent* in the Greek New Testament simply means, "to turn around."[1] It was once a military term that described a soldier marching in one direction and then doing an about-face. When this word is used in the spiritual sense, it means to change your mind.

Today, you have been given a choice—a new chance. Yesterday and its failures are gone and a thing of the past. Today, you have the ability to create your tomorrow.

> Yesterday and its failures are gone and
> a thing of the past. Today, you have
> the ability to create your tomorrow.

Body

Take out a notecard or a journal. I want you to think about what your life could look like in five years if you made the choice to choose health today. On the back of it, write out what your life could look like in five years.

Soul

We all have the ability to choose whether we want to live in the past or move forward into the future.

Spirit

God, I come before You and I repent for believing the lie that I cannot change. Please help guide me as I continually renew my mind and align my thoughts with Yours.

Note

1. John J. Parsons, "Thoughts about Repentance: Teshuvah, Metanoia, and Strepho," Hebrew for Christians, accessed June 25, 2016, http://www.hebrew4christians.com/Holidays/Fall_Holidays/Elul/Teshuvah/teshuvah.html.

LETTING GO OF CONTROL

You will keep in perfect peace those whose
minds are steadfast, because they trust in you.
—ISAIAH 26:3 NIV

Oftentimes life can feel like a balancing act. We juggle everything—our jobs, children, marriages, as well as social obligations such as church events or school productions. We sometimes go through our days just trying to keep everyone and everything from falling part. The pressure is overwhelming, and we find ourselves ending our day with our head to the pillow replaying everything that didn't get done and every moment when we maybe didn't act our best. We drift off to sleep, embarrassed or ashamed at our own lack.

If you have found yourself in a similar situation, I have good news for you. We weren't created to be able to do it all. Oftentimes that statement isn't shocking because we all know better than to believe that we can juggle it all, yet we still try to be the one who exceeds everyone's expectations. This will lead to burnout and even maybe resentment toward our loved ones.

Learning to let go of control and the need to be perceived as perfect is one of the greatest lessons that many of us have yet to learn. The need for control and perfectionism is often due to the fact that we have begun to find our identity in those things. When we do this, we have only set ourselves up for failure and disappointment.

Reinhold Niebuhr, who penned "The Serenity Prayer," prayed, "God, grant me the serenity to accept the things I cannot change, the courage to change the things I can, and the wisdom to know the difference." Many of us can benefit by allowing the words of this simple prayer to wash over us. Once we give ourselves permission to not be everything for everyone, we will once again find our peace within God.

> We all know better than to believe that we can juggle it all, yet we all still try to be the one who exceeds everyone's expectations.

Body

Throughout your day, I want you to take an honest account of how many times you beat yourself up for not being enough. When the lie that you are not enough enters your mind, take a moment and declare the truth over yourself that just as you are, you are enough.

Soul

Perfectionism can be deadly disease. It sucks the life out of us and leaves us feeling small and obsolete. The truth is that we were never created to be perfect.

Spirit

Father, I thank You that You have never expected me to be perfect. Thank You for Your grace and the ability to take one day at a time with You alongside me. Please help me extend grace to myself in the process and show me all the ways I am victorious.

THE JOY OF THE LORD

You make known to me the path of life; you
will fill me with joy in your presence, with
eternal pleasures at your right hand.
—PSALM 16:11 NIV

One of my favorite fruits of the Spirit is joy. I truly believe that joy is essential to the human experience and for good soul health. Have you ever stopped to watch children play? They laugh without fear because they have found what it is like to experience true joy! Proverbs 17:22 says, "A joyful heart is good medicine, but a crushed spirit dries up the bones" (ESV).

There are many of us who may have lost our joy. Circumstances in life can try to rob us of the gift of joy. The loss of a job, the passing of a loved one, divorce, and sickness can all try to take us under in waves of grief and heartache. In these seasons, it's important to remember that just because we feel we have lost our joy, God hasn't lost His! Nehemiah 8:10 says, "Don't be dejected and sad, for the joy of the Lord is your strength!" (NLT).

There is a reason that it's His joy that is our strength! God could have used any other attribute—His love, His peace, or His gentleness—but instead He chooses to give us His joy to lean on. It's what weaves the moments of our lives together and helps us press forward in the dark times while building momentum in the good times.

Today, I encourage you to be brave enough to find your joy again! If you have a hard time feeling joyful, don't be afraid to allow yourself to rest; watch good, clean, funny movies and begin to appreciate laughter.

Joy weaves the moments of our lives together and helps us press forward in the dark times while building momentum in the good times.

Body

Take out a journal and list the things that have tried to steal your joy. When you are done, ask the Holy Spirit to show you where the joy in those situations hides.

Soul

Joy is the wellspring of life. It is what helps us get through every day. Having joy means you have the ability to stand against anything that the enemy tries to throw against you.

Spirit

Father, I thank You for giving me Your joy! I lay before You the things that have tried to steal my joy and I ask that You replace the heartache with Your joy. Thank You that Your joy is a promise that I can grab hold of!

DECLARE THE TRUTH

May these words of my mouth and this
meditation of my heart be pleasing in your
sight, Lord, my Rock and my Redeemer.
—PSALM 19:14 NIV

Declarations have been a powerful source in my life as well as the lives of others. Declarations are a God-given tool because they release the power of the spoken word over lives, our relationships, our situations, and ourselves.

Proverbs 18:21 says, "Death and life are in the power of the tongue" (KJV). What a powerful statement! In the story of creation, we see that God used words to create the universe. In the same storyline, we learned that when God created man, He created us in His image. I believe that when He did this, He also gave us the ability to create our own worlds with our words.

Many of us are guilty of using our words negatively, especially against ourselves. Have you ever heard the words spoken in a women's dressing room? *"I'm so fat…I'll never lose weight…I'll never find a boyfriend with these love handles."* If we consider the power that our words carry, those statements become terrifying!

We were made to communicate with words. When we speak, our mind, body, and spirit all are called to attention. This is why it is extremely important that our words are life-giving and full of promise! A great way to find some good declarations is to simply ask God how He sees you. What does He love about you? What does He have in store for you? Once we know how God sees us, we can begin to align our minds, healing our souls, by speaking forth those truths.

> When we speak, our mind, body, and spirit all are called to attention.

Body

Take out a journal and ask God to give you five declarations that He wants you to begin declaring over yourself. Write those declarations down and keep them in a place where you will remember to look at them every day. Challenge yourself to say them once, twice, or even three times a day! Really allow these truths to be saturated into your spirit.

Soul

Our words have power! When we speak, the world around us listens. Speaking forth the promises and goodness of God will help shape our destiny.

Spirit

Father, I repent for using my own words against myself. I thank You that You have given me the power to shape the world around me. May my words be uplifting to You, myself, and to others.

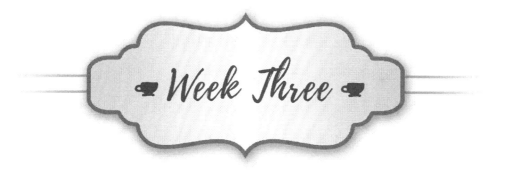

Week Three

CELEBRATING THE TRIUNE CONNECTION

Now may the God of peace himself sanctify
you completely, and may your whole spirit
and soul and body be kept blameless at
the coming of our Lord Jesus Christ.
—1 THESSALONIANS 5:23 ESV

I love nature. I've always been fascinated with the world around me and I feel the Lord when I look at His intricate creation. The vast glory of the mountains, the deep mystery of the ocean, the peaceful flow of a strong river: They all showcase the wonder and the majesty of God. What I find even more fascinating is that as beautiful as all those things are, they are not even His greatest creation. We are.

When God created the world, He made the decision to make man in His own image. Wow! God, in His sovereignty, knew that we would fall short, but He decided that we were still worth the risk. His love for us runs so deep.

God is a triune being—the Father, the Son, and the Holy Spirit. They are three separate entities and yet one. Just as He is three in one, He gave us three beings as well. Our bodies, our souls, and our spirits. Each is fully different but they all work together to create who we actually are. They are all of equal importance, and we are responsible for stewarding them fully.

In First Thessalonians 5:23, the apostle Paul writes, "Now may the God of peace Himself sanctify you entirely; and may your *spirit* and *soul* and *body* be preserved complete, without blame at the coming of our Lord Jesus Christ" (NASB). This verse shows that each of our beings are of value to God.

In our culture, we have a tendency to focus most of our attention toward only one aspect of who we are. Some people are so entirely focused on their physical bodies that they neglect their spirituality, while others are so focused on their spirit life that they forget to renew their minds or to steward their physical bodies. I encourage you to begin seeing yourself in a new perspective; fully embrace that you are made up of three parts and each deserves your love and attention.

God, in His sovereignty, knew that
we would fall short, but He decided
that we were still worth the risk.

Body

Today, I want you to be intentional about getting to fully know yourself. Open your journal and allow yourself to have a few minutes in peace. Focus on how your body feels. What would it say to you if it could speak? How does your mind feel? Is it restless? Excited? How does your spirit feel? Does it feel tired or alive? Journal your thoughts and revelations and ask the Lord to give you direction when it comes to your three beings.

Soul

Just as God is made of three parts, we are also made up of a triune being. Our body, soul, and spirit all make up who we are, and it is important that we treat each part of us with love and kindness.

Spirit

Father, I thank You that You chose to make me in Your image! I ask that as I explore getting to know every part of me, You meet me in this process. I give You permission to show me ways in which I can grow and also to show me the things that You love about each part of me.

THE BODY AND SOUL CONNECTION

The eye is the lamp of the body. If your eyes are
healthy, your whole body will be full of light.
—MATTHEW 6:22 NIV

One of my greatest joys is being able to travel to different churches. Being able to meet and teach others who are part of the Body of Christ is an honor that I do not take for granted. In 2009, my husband and I had both been traveling quite a lot for a few years. At that point, my body began to become tired, and I knew that I had to slow down and take better care of myself.

I was overworked, tired, and just not feeling like myself. Over the course of the next few months, I began to rest and spend a lot of my time in worship and communion with God. During this time, I met with a friend who introduced me to something called an "invisible clock." At the time, she had been dealing with various health issues, and her doctor had his patients wear this product. She had it set to vibrate every 10 to 20 minutes, and when it did it would remind her to pause and give thanks to God. I almost immediately purchased one for myself and began wearing it daily. After about three weeks, I woke up one morning and my overall being felt more alive! I realized that when I began focusing on aligning my soul and my spirit with God, my body soon followed suit!

This story beautifully illustrates just how connected we are. When our minds or our spirits are unhealthy, our bodies may begin to feel run down or sick. To be clear, I am not saying that those who are physically sick have unhealthy souls or spirits. I am just sharing my own testimony of how my being was fully connected.

If you are feeling tired, I encourage you to spend some time aligning yourself with God in worship and thanksgiving!

> When I began focusing on aligning
> my soul and my spirit with God,
> my body soon followed suit!

Body

Take some time to fully experience God in your body, soul, and spirit. Take a moment to sit in stillness and take an account for how you feel. How does your body feel? Tired? Run down? Calm? Next move on to your mind. Do you feel anxious or at peace? How does your spirit feel? Do you feel connected to God? Write down what you discover about yourself and ask the Holy Spirit to help you be more aware of how each of your beings connects with the others.

Soul

We are a triune being! Each part of our nature was intended to help the other. When one part of us is sick, it may manifest in a different part. Being able to steward ourselves means being able to be aware of what is going on in each part of us.

Spirit

Father, I thank You that You have made me wonderfully complex! Please help me become more aware of my body, my soul, and my spirit. Give me the wisdom I need when I can sense that something is off and help me be a good steward of myself.

FIGHTING YOUR GOLIATH

And God raised the Lord and will
also raise us up by his power.
—1 CORINTHIANS 6:14 ESV

I love the story of David and Goliath because it is a story of a young boy who defied all odds and did the impossible. David was just a young boy from Bethlehem and the youngest of four boys. While his older brothers were part of the Israelite army, David stayed home and tended to his father's sheep. When a Philistine giant began to threaten the Israelites, the community and soldiers cowered in fear. There was even a great reward issued from the king for anyone who could kill off this giant.

David was the least likely person to be able to attempt such a feat. In fact, he was mocked when people found out that he wanted to try to take down Goliath. However, David didn't let other people's doubts and words stop him from fully pressing on.

Courage and one smooth stone was all it took to take down Goliath. Physically, David should not have been able to take down such a giant. However, his spirit believed in who God created him to be and he aligned his mind with this belief. This allowed him to fight Goliath!

What is your Goliath? Maybe it's this very journey of health that you are on. Maybe it's a job, a relationship, or a financial hardship. I encourage you to look at David as an example of someone who didn't have what it took on his own, but when he aligned his mind, body, and spirit with the Lord, it gave him a supernatural ability to fight Goliath. God will do the same for you; you only need to be willing to stand up to fight.

His spirit believed in who God created him to be and he aligned his mind with this belief.

Body

Make a list of your three greatest fears. Journal about why you feel afraid to go after those areas in your life. Then I want you to journal what it would look like if God intervened in the way only He can.

Soul

Life has its own set of giants, and oftentimes we can run in fear of them. However, we've been made to be able to conquer them in body, soul, and spirit.

Spirit

Father, I thank You for the gift of supernatural increase when I partner with You! I thank You that I was not created to live in fear but to live in victory! I ask that You stand beside me as I learn to look my fear in the face and push toward victory!

WHERE YOUR EMOTIONS RESIDE

Finally, be strong in the Lord and
in the strength of his might.
—EPHESIANS 6:10 ESV

I have a friend who was going through a difficult season in her life. In a short period of time, she lost two very close family members. The first month after her losses, she was able to go about her life just the same and kept herself distracted and busy. She was avoiding having to feel the pain of losing her loved ones. Her method seemed to be working until a few weeks had passed. Suddenly, she began experiencing panic attacks and extreme insomnia to the point of only sleeping a few broken up hours a night. She became depressed, lethargic, and overall exhausted from the lack of sleep and constant fits of anxiety.

She eventually came to me asking for advice and was desperate enough to try anything. I told her she needed to first allow herself to grieve and actually feel the pain that she had been avoiding and then, second, take time to soak in the Lord's presence. She took my advice and was amazed that within just a few short weeks, her panic attacks subsided completely!

This is a wonderful example of just how connected our whole being is. Her spirit was in pain and grieved after experiencing the trauma of death, but because her mind did not want to allow her to feel the pain it eventually began to manifest physically in her body, which caused her panic attacks. Once she paid attention to what was going on inside of her heart, her physical pain began to subside.

Proverbs 13:12 tells us that "hope deferred makes the heart sick" (NIV). This tells us that whatever is going on inside of our soul or spirit has the ability to affect our physical body. I encourage you to pay closer attention to what may be stirring within your heart. Don't be afraid to allow yourself to feel pain, however uncomfortable it may be, and know that the Holy Spirit will be there to comfort you in the process.

> Whatever is going on inside of
> our soul or spirit has the ability
> to affect our physical body.

Body

Take a moment to take inventory of your heart. What is it feeling? What emotions come to mind when you focus on it?

Take a few moments and journal what emotions are brought to your attention. Sometimes it is even helpful to ask your heart what it is feeling. Focus on giving your heart a voice this week and pay attention to it.

Soul

Our emotions are there to communicate with us. Uncomfortable emotions such as pain, sadness, and fear can be scary and unnerving. But the only thing scarier than allowing ourselves to feel pain is what will happen when we run from it.

Spirit

Father, I thank You for the gift of emotions. I ask that You stand by my side and help me be unafraid of pain. I ask that in the moments when I am tempted to run, You hold my hand and be my source of strength.

RESPECTING THE ARTIST

So God created mankind in his own image,
in the image of God he created them;
male and female he created them.
—GENESIS 1:27 NIV

One of my favorite parts about being able to travel to different parts of the world is being able to enjoy the different cultures. I love seeing how different cultures celebrate beauty, music, and art in their own ways. My husband and I love collecting portraits and paintings from all over the world and putting them up for display in our home. Naturally, when a large price is paid for something, you do everything in your power to make sure the art piece is taken care of and does not become dirty or broken. If I were to purchase an expensive piece of art and immediately become careless and drop it in front of the artist, it would bring great disdain and offense to the artist.

We should be viewing our body, soul, and spirit in just the same way. Psalm 139:13 tells us that God carefully knit us together in our mother's womb. He carefully constructed every detail from the hairs on our head to our personality traits. He knows and formed every detail of us, which only shows how vast his love for us is. We are His work of art, His masterpiece.

When I had this revelation, I decided that I didn't want to grieve the great artist by not taking care of and being a poor steward of my body. As hard as it can be to stay on the journey of health, the price for wavering is even greater. I encourage you to begin seeing your body as a piece of art designed by the great creator himself! You are of so much value, and my prayer for you is that you begin to truly see your worth.

We are His work of art, His masterpiece.

Body

Take a few minutes and really think about each part of your body. Your arms, your stomach, and your legs. In your journal, I want you to write three things that you love and appreciate about each part of your body. This will help shift your focus from the negative things you may dislike to the positive things that your body does for you on a daily basis.

Soul

When we stop to realize that God put much attention and detail into creating us, it makes us appreciate ourselves and our bodies more! When we speak negatively about ourselves, we are speaking negatively about something God created. Learning to appreciate ourselves and our bodies brings honor to God.

Spirit

Father, I thank You for making me just as I am! I repent for the negative words or thoughts I have had toward my body, and Please help me relearn how to love and appreciate the body and mind that You have created for me.

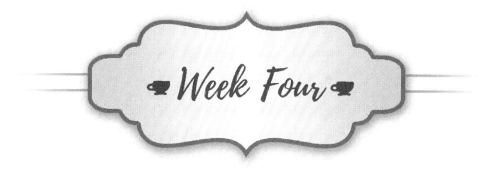

Week Four

THE POWER OF REST

By the seventh day God had finished the work he
had been doing; so on the seventh day he rested
from all his work. Then God blessed the seventh
day and made it holy, because on it he rested
from all the work of creating that he had done.
—GENESIS 2:2-3 NIV

I am very blessed to be able to live the life that I do. When the
Lord moved at Bethel, our lives were forever changed both on
a spiritual and practical level. At one point, both my husband
and I were traveling numerous times throughout the year. At
first it was exciting because I love being able to minister and
meet new people in the church. However, I never took my own
need for rest into consideration, and after a while I began to feel
both physically and mentally exhausted. I remember looking

at my assistant during an international flight home saying, "I don't think I can do this anymore."

My body had been tired for a long time, and eventually it led to mental exhaustion. I went to my doctor and was given strict orders—*rest*. The next few months were committed to getting well by allowing myself to sleep, relax, and laugh. Over time, my body began to heal, which allowed for me to once again feel like myself.

One of the greatest examples of the need to rest comes from God Himself! In Genesis 1, we read about the creation of the world. Everything that we know and see was created over a period of six days. God could have ended the story of creation after chapter one; however, He continues into chapter two where we read about the most mysterious part of creation. God rested. Why would God have a need to rest? I don't feel inclined to believe that He really needed a long nap or to catch up on His favorite television shows. No, He rested because He wanted to show us the importance of rest.

Rest allows for us to bring realignment to our body, soul, and spirit. Our physical bodies grow weary, our souls can become cluttered, and our spirits grow hungry if we go without rest. God, in His loving kindness, knew that this would be the case for us. So He set the example to show us the importance of rest.

Many of us lead busy lives. Many people have asked me—between work, family, friends, and social obligations, who can find the time for rest? My question is, who can find the time for burnout? In the long run, everyone, including yourself, is going to benefit deeply from your ability to love yourself enough to rest.

> Who can find the time for rest? Who
> can find the time for burnout?

Body

Resting is a form of self-love. Today, I want you to schedule a time this week to make it a point to rest. Rest doesn't have to look like sleeping; however, please feel free to do so! Rest can look like anything that helps you relax, whether it's a long walk, journaling, taking a bath, or reading a book. Be intentional and schedule an appointment with yourself to rest!

Soul

We were not created to live off of adrenaline. Resting is a form of worship to God because we are following His example and command. Giving yourself permission to rest is one of the greatest forms of self-love.

Spirit

Father, I thank You that You are always the ultimate example for me. Please help lead me as I learn to allow myself to rest. I trust that by doing so, my relationships with myself, my family, and with You will flourish and grow stronger.

RESTING IN THE PRESENCE OF JESUS

> The Lord is my shepherd, I lack nothing. He
> makes me lie down in green pastures, he leads
> me beside quiet waters, he refreshes my soul.
> —PSALM 23:1-3 NIV

A beautiful story in the Bible is the story of Mary and Martha. Mary and Martha were dear friends and faithful followers of Jesus. I imagine the two sisters to be full of life and known for their adoration for the Lord. In Luke 10, we read of the time when Jesus paid a visit to their home.

> *As Jesus and the disciples continued on their way to Jeru-*
> *salem, they came to a certain village where a woman*
> *named Martha welcomed him into her home. Her sister,*
> *Mary, sat at the Lord's feet, listening to what he taught.*
> *But Martha was distracted by the big dinner she was*

preparing. She came to Jesus and said, "Lord, doesn't it seem unfair to you that my sister just sits here while I do all the work? Tell her to come and help me."

But the Lord said to her, "My dear Martha, you are worried and upset over all these details! There is only one thing worth being concerned about. Mary has discovered it, and it will not be taken away from her" (Luke 10:38–42 NLT).

My guess is that Martha was given the gift of hospitality! We can see how, when Jesus arrived, her focus was on her work. She wanted everything just right. The food freshly prepared, the house clean, the table set, and the atmosphere welcoming. She became so wrapped up in the presentation that she began to miss out on the gift she was being given in the moment— Jesus, a guest in her own home!

I think that we can all relate to Martha. The pressures to look a certain way, be a certain way, or live a certain life can cause us to lose sight of what is really important. Mary, on the other hand, recognized the gift that she had access to. She didn't care what the world said she needed to be doing; all she cared about was being in the presence of Jesus.

Let's not get so caught up in our own lives that we miss Jesus in the room. I pray that we all become a Mary and learn to rest in the presence and grace of Christ.

> Let's not get so caught up in our own
> lives that we miss Jesus in the room.

Body

Today your assignment is easy—rest in Jesus. Take a few moments to really connect with His presence. I encourage you to lay aside any questions or prayers you may have and just allow yourself to sit in His presence and goodness.

Soul

Learning to rest in Jesus will become one of our greatest strengths. It's in the seasons of rest that we learn how to fight the battles we come across.

Spirit

Jesus, it is my heart's desire to sit at Your feet because there is where the hope of my heart lies. I ask that You give me a heart like Mary, one that knows how to rest in Your presence.

RESTING IS A FORM OF TRUST

You will keep in perfect peace those whose
minds are steadfast, because they trust in you.
—ISAIAH 26:3 NIV

Many of us have experienced a sleepless night. Your body is tired but your mind is racing. You lie awake as you watch the clock tick later and later into the night. Fear and anxiety begin to creep in as your mind races through every unfortunate scenario that could possibly happen to you. Maybe it's finances, a troubled child, a hurting marriage, or a sick friend or family member. Whatever it is, your mind can't seem to release it to God.

Sleep in itself can be a very vulnerable thing. When we are asleep, we forfeit our control. We willingly become unaware of the world around us, which can be extremely scary for some. The need for control is a paralyzing condition for many. Having control can make us feel powerful, so the thought of losing it makes us feel powerless.

As Christians, we can sleep at peace knowing that the Lord never sleeps. Psalm 121:3–6 says, "He will not let you stumble; the one who watches over you will not slumber. Indeed, he who watches over Israel never slumbers or sleeps. The Lord himself watches over you! The Lord stands beside you as your protective shade. The sun will not harm you by day, nor the moon at night" (NLT).

The Lord, who watches over us, never sleeps or slumbers! This verse gives me great peace, as I lay my head to my pillow, because I know that I can trust Him to take care of me even while I sleep. Fear and anxiety may try to pollute my mind, but I know that my God is bigger than any problem I may be facing!

Jesus Himself can provide a wonderful example of this. In Matthew 8, we see Jesus and His disciples on a boat. While Jesus was asleep, a great storm began to overtake the boat, leaving the disciples frightened and worried. They awakened Jesus in a panic and Jesus simply woke up, rebuked the winds, and accused His disciples of having no faith. I am sure the disciples were stunned by His words because they surely thought they were not going to make it out of that boat alive! But Jesus stayed in peace and rest, which gave Him authority over the winds.

I know that we all go through difficult seasons and find ourselves unable to rest, but I encourage you to begin to surrender your anxiety and fear before the Lord. He will grant you great rest.

Begin to surrender your anxiety and fear
before the Lord. He will grant you great rest.

Body

As you prepare for bed this evening, I want you to make a conscious effort to quiet your mind and lay before the Lord anything that is heavy on your heart. Sometimes it helps to read a scripture and to fall asleep with the scripture in my mind or to repeat "I trust you, Jesus" every time fear or anxiety may try to creep in. Whatever you find helps, I encourage you to be intentional about letting go of control and receiving His peace.

Soul

When we learn to rest, we actually are honoring God by showing that we have placed our trust in Him.

Spirit

*Father, I thank You that in You I find a place of refuge.
I release to You any fear, anxiety, or control that I have
tried to hold on to and I openly receive Your blessing and
peace in return.*

LIVING WATER

But whoever drinks of the water that I will
give him shall never thirst; but the water
that I will give him will become in him a well
of water springing up to eternal life.
—JOHN 4:14 NASB

Throughout the Bible, we see illustration upon illustration of water. In John 7, Jesus famously referred to Himself as the "living water," inviting all who were thirsty to come to Him where they will never thirst again. In the Psalms, King David cried out to God saying, "My soul thirsts for you; my whole body longs for you in this parched and weary land where there is no water" (Ps. 63:1 NLT). Again, in the book of Revelation John has a vision of the Lord saying, "The Spirit and the bride say, 'Come.' Let anyone who hears this say, 'Come.' Let anyone who is thirsty come. Let anyone who desires drink freely from the water of life" (Rev. 22:17 NLT).

As you can see, water is used time and time again throughout the Bible as an illustration for the source of life. One thing that I love about God is that He often uses things that are true in the natural to show us truth in the spiritual! Living water is not only essential for our souls and spirits, but it is of vital importance for our physical bodies as well.

The human body can go weeks or even months without food or nutrition, but it can only survive a few days without water.[1] Wow! Water is the cash flow of the body, meaning it is what keeps our bodies alive and able to function.[2] Keeping hydrated is just one of many ways that we steward our bodies that we have been given.

I encourage you to not only allow yourself to be immersed in living water but to also not forget about your physical body as well. Both are of great importance to God and we will reap lasting benefits.

> Living water is not only essential for our souls and spirits, but it is of vital importance for our physical bodies as well.

Body

I want you to set a goal for yourself for today both spiritually and physically. On the physical goal, make sure you keep hydrated! Make a goal to drink at least eight glasses of water today. On the spiritual side, allow yourself to experience God as the living water. If there is a situation you are facing or a belief system that you want to conquer, ask the Lord to pour His living water upon you to give you greater clarity and guidance.

Soul

The Bible uses water to explain the importance of God for our soul and spirit! In the same way, physical water is vital to our bodies. Keeping hydrated will allow us to experience God fully in body, soul, and spirit.

Spirit

Father, I thank You for Your living water! I am forever grateful that I can go to You and never thirst again. I thank You for the gift of water and the ability to hydrate my body and the gift of Your living water. Please help me to never take for granted what You have provided for me both spiritually and physically.

Notes

1. Dina Spector, "Here's How Many Days a Person Can Survive Without Water," Business Insider, May 09, 2014, http://www.businessinsider.com/how-many-days-can-you-survive-without-water-2014-5.
2. Beni Johnson and Jordan Rubin, *Healthy and Free* (Shippensburg, PA: Destiny Image Publishers, 2015), 53.

WATER BRINGS LIFE

Then the angel showed me a river with the
water of life, clear as crystal, flowing from
the throne of God and of the Lamb.
—REVELATION 22:1 NLT

Throughout the Bible, water plays a vital role in many stories. In Scripture, we can see how water was actually the foundation for breakthrough and miracles to be birthed. Here are just a few examples.

In Genesis, we see that before the earth was formed, it was just dark water. Out of the water came land and life as God called it forth.

Noah was commanded to build a boat to save himself and his family from the flood. The flood represented the end of an evil era and the human race having a second chance at life.

In Exodus, Moses began leading the Israelites out of slavery and into the Promised Land. The Egyptians came after them to lead them back into captivity, but God parted the waters of the Red Sea, which provided an escape for the Israelites.

In John, we read about Jesus' first miracle of turning water into wine while at a wedding. The water became the foundation to create that miracle, which in turn led to the revelation of who Jesus truly was.

In John, Jesus approached a Samaritan woman who was drawing water from the city well. When He asked her for a drink of water, He was breaking tradition because Jews did not associate with Samaritans, especially a woman. This moment in time broke down the cultural walls and the oppression that women had to endure.

As we can see, water was used to help bring forth life, breakthrough, and miracles. The same is true in the physical realm. In my book, I tell the story of a friend who came to me because her mom was sick. The doctors were unable to find anything wrong with her after numerous tests. I advised her to have her mom begin drinking water and to check back with me in a few weeks. After a few weeks, she was happy to report that her mom was no longer sick! Just adding water cured what could have cost them hundreds in medical bills and tests!

God knew what He was doing when He gave us the gift of water. Water is the birthplace of life, healing, and wholeness! May we be forever grateful that we have been given such a gift.

God knew what He was doing when He gave us the gift of water. Water is the birthplace of life, healing, and wholeness!

Body

Is there an area in your life that feels dead? Maybe it's a dream that you let die after encountering fear or failure or maybe it's a relationship that needs new life breathed upon it. God promises to bring hope and life to every area of our lives! Get before God and ask Him to pour His living water upon whichever area is highlighted to you. Ask Him to give you new perspective, ideas, or hope for those areas. In a journal, write what He says to you.

Soul

Water, in its history, has been the birthplace for life, miracles, and breakthrough. Just the simple task of keeping hydrated allows us to experience the miracle of life on a daily basis.

Spirit

Father, I thank for the life and the breakthrough that water has brought throughout history. I ask that as I learn to properly hydrate in both the spiritual and the physical realms, You will release the same breakthrough to me.

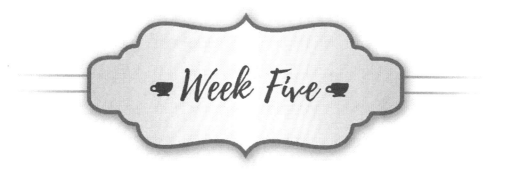

Week Five

FINDING THE COURAGE

Finally, be strong in the Lord and
in the strength of his might.
—EPHESIANS 6:10 ESV

In life, we are forced to do things that we don't necessarily want to do. Pay bills, run errands, report to jury duty, and everyone's favorite—exercise.

Ugh. Even the word alone is enough to make some people cringe! Visions of hours dedicated to a treadmill while gasping for air come to their minds. The problem is that people tend to view exercise as a form of punishment instead of as a key to lasting health! Oftentimes, when it comes to adding anything new in life, the hardest part is just getting started. The thought of something new or unfamiliar is often scarier than the thing itself. It takes a certain kind of courage to take the first step forward.

Abraham stands as an example of someone who had to be willing to face change head-on in order to receive the promises that the Lord had for him. In Genesis 12, God said:

> *Leave your native country, your relatives, and your father's family, and go to the land that I will show you. I will make you into a great nation. I will bless you and make you famous, and you will be a blessing to others* (Genesis 12:1-2 NLT).

In those times, family was a source of identity. Leaving one's own family was not common and surely would take a huge step of faith. When the Lord asked Abraham to leave his father's family, Abraham had to make a choice. Was he willing to take that leap of faith and believe that God had something better in store for him even if that meant risking leaving everything that he knew behind? Or would he allow fear to dictate his choices and keep him from ever knowing or experiencing the fullness of the destiny ahead for him? Thankfully, Abraham chose to trust God, and his decision is still affecting us thousands of years later.

Incorporating any sort of change can always be scary. Exercise is often intimidating, and many of us never take the first step toward trying it because we have already convinced ourselves that we are going to fail. I encourage you to not allow fear to dictate your life anymore. Yes, it will be hard. There will be days when the thought of hiding in bed with a box of donuts is going to sound more tempting than lifting weights, but I promise you that the small sacrifice of doing something you are afraid to do is going to far outweigh the temporary satisfaction of sitting at home.

*The only thing scarier than change
is not changing at all.*

Body

Take out our journal, and I want you to list five ways that your life would look differently if you found the courage to begin exercising. I also want you to imagine how your life would be different six months and one year from now if you continued your exercise regimen. Imagine how you would feel and what goals you would be proud of.

Soul

Change is scary. But the only thing scarier than change is not changing at all. Find the courage within yourself to be willing to take the first step toward lasting change.

Spirit

Father, I thank You that I have this opportunity to add exercise to my life. I thank You for giving me the strength and the ability to take this first step toward change. Please give me strength in my moments of weakness and courage in the moments when I doubt myself.

DEFINING SUCCESS

I can do all this through him who gives me strength.
—PHILIPPIANS 4:13 NIV

Many of us have been there. It's 2 a.m., and for whatever reason we just cannot drift off into sleep. Maybe it's stress or maybe it was due to a few too many coffees in the day, but whatever it is it forces us to get up and wander to the living room where were turn on the TV. At that time of night, infomercials plague our TV screens and many of them are targeted toward those of us who want to lose weight. Toned abs, legs, and arms flash across the screen and they show us before and after photos. After seeing messages like that, it's easy to give in to the belief that we are only truly successful if we look like the people do on TV or in magazines.

By now, many of us know that the journey toward health looks different on everybody. No one has the same body shape or body chemistry and makeup, so why are we expected to look like they do in magazines?

Galatians 6:4 tells us, "Let everyone be sure that he is doing his very best, for then he will have the personal satisfaction of work well done and won't need to compare himself with someone else" (TLB). I love this verse because it can be applied in so many areas of our lives. When we begin an exercise program, it is easy to become discouraged when we don't see immediate results or when we begin comparing our results and progress with others. However, when we do that we begin to belittle the benefits that our efforts have had on both our body and our minds.

I encourage you to find what your own definition of success is when it comes to exercise. Maybe success looks like taking a brisk walk when you felt like staying in bed or doing some sit ups in between the kids' nap times. Whatever it is, learn to celebrate your success without comparing yourself to others! This is your journey and you deserve to feel victorious!

No one has the same body shape or body chemistry and makeup, so why are we expected to look like they do in magazines?

Body

Take a moment to think about what your goals are realistically. Write at least three goals you have for yourself in a journal along with a plan of action that will help get you to those goals. If you're afraid that you are being too unrealistic or too easy on yourself, share your goals with a friend who can give you encouraging feedback.

Soul

We were not designed to look like everyone else! Our journeys are all different and the most important aspect of health is making sure we take the path that is the healthiest for us.

Spirit

Father, I thank You that I am not expected to do this journey perfectly. Please help me give myself grace as I learn more about my body and learn about the wisest path for me to take. Thank You for being my faithful guide!

THE TEMPLE OF GOD

Therefore, I urge you, brothers and sisters, in
view of God's mercy, to offer your bodies as
a living sacrifice, holy and pleasing to God—
this is your true and proper worship.
—ROMANS 12:1 NIV

I remember being a young mom with three young children running around the house. Children have a tendency to make a mess of things by leaving toys scattered about and shoes, clothing, and dishes in unexpected places. I did my best to keep tidy after them, but let's be honest—it is almost impossible to keep a house clean at all times especially with children. However, if I knew that an important guest was going to be coming over and staying with us, I would go out of my way to make sure my house was not only presentable but also enjoyable to be in! The dishes would be done, the bathrooms would be scrubbed clean, and my children's toys would be in their rooms. I would want my guest of honor to feel comfortable in my home!

The same is true for our bodies. In First Corinthians 6:19 it says, "Do you not know that your bodies are temples of the Holy Spirit, who is in you, whom you have received from God? You are not your own" (NIV). Our bodies were made to be the dwelling place of God. Wow! Stop and think about that for a second. He could have chosen to make His home any place in the world, but His desire was to be as close to us as possible. When we don't take care of our bodies, we are destroying the home of God.

As you go about your day today, stop and think about how you are stewarding the temple of the Lord. Are your choices lining up with how you would want His home to be, or are they making it a less enjoyable place to stay? I can guarantee that as you choose to honor your body with good food and exercise not only are you honoring yourself, but also you are honoring the Lord.

As you choose to honor your body with good food and exercise not only are you honoring yourself, but also you are honoring the Lord.

Body

Now that we know that our bodies are the temple of God, it is important that we learn to care for them. In your journal, write out in as much detail as you can what a healthy body for God to reside in would look like. What changes do you have to make to be sure that you can provide a healthy and welcoming environment for God?

Soul

Our bodies are the temple of God! It is an honor to be able to steward a home for our King, and it is our responsibility to care for it.

Spirit

Father, I thank You that You have made my body Your home. Please continue to remind me that taking care of my body is not only for my benefit but for Yours. Thank You for the opportunity to be able to be Your resting place.

PRESSING ON TOWARD THE GOAL

I press on toward the goal to win the prize for which
God has called me heavenward in Christ Jesus.
—PHILIPPIANS 3:14 NIV

The most common phrase I hear when I encourage someone to begin working out is, "I hate exercise!" Let's be honest, we've all groaned at one point at the thought of having to force ourselves out of the house and log yet another mile on the treadmill. Sometimes making yourself move just isn't fun! However, part of maturity is accepting that sometimes we have to do things that we don't want to do in order to serve the bigger picture.

Hebrews 12:11 tells us that, "No discipline seems pleasant at the time, but painful. Later on, however, it produces a harvest of righteousness and peace for those who have been trained by it" (NIV). I love that it says that it gives us "a *peace* for those who have been trained by it" because it shows that there is always a good reward when we are willing to step outside of our comfort zone and be diligent.

We live in a culture where we are naturally drawn to fast results. This mindset can be extremely harmful, especially when applied to a journey like health and wellness. Long-lasting results often take time, patience, and diligence. Obstacles and mistakes are inevitable in this journey, but like Paul says in Philippians 3:14, we are called to "press on toward the goal to win the prize for which God has called me heavenward in Christ Jesus."

I encourage you today that if you feel unmotivated or afraid to take the next step, allow yourself to see the bigger picture. Feel encouraged knowing that if you allow yourself to be disciplined now, you will soon be walking in the peace it will bring in the future.

> There is always a good reward when we are willing to step outside of our comfort zone and be diligent.

Body

Today, your goal is to make yourself do something that you don't want to do, knowing that you will reap the rewards! Whether it's 50 jumping jacks, a brisk walk, or an at-home

DVD, set your goal and discipline yourself to make sure you accomplish it.

Soul

Exercise, like any other discipline, may not feel good in the moment; however, we can rest knowing that we will someday walk in its fruits. In those moments when you feel like skipping a workout or quitting early, remind yourself of your "Why" and be motivated knowing that you will someday reap its rewards!

Spirit

Father, I thank You for the gift of discipline and I pray that You give me a heart for receiving it. Please continue to remind me of the fruit that I will receive when I push past my comfort zone and allow myself to be stretched.

UNENDING GRACE

But he said to me, "My grace is sufficient for you,
for my power is made perfect in weakness."
—2 CORINTHIANS 12:9 ESV

A mistake that many people make when they begin incorporating exercise into their lives is trying to tackle too much at one time. We may dream of being the greatest athlete, the fastest runner, or the strongest person in the weight room, but we have to allow ourselves time to get there.

The Bible is filled with stories of people who in the natural didn't have what it takes, but when they partnered with God they were able to do the impossible. Moses was a man who had a speech impediment, yet God called him to speak in front of the most powerful man in Egypt at the time! David was just a shepherd who was faithful in tending to his father's sheep, and God used him to defeat Goliath. Mary was just a young unmarried girl who held no social significance in her culture, yet God used her to birth His Son into this world.

You see, sometimes when we look at our dreams or hopes for our future, it is easy to partner with the thoughts of defeat. We think that we are too heavy to ever be able to run a marathon, too sick to ever feel well enough to exercise, too damaged to ever feel significant again. But God says otherwise! In Matthew 19:26 we hear Jesus say, "With man this is impossible, but with God all things are possible" (NIV). If we really allow those words to sink into our hearts, we will realize the weight and the power that they carry!

I encourage you to extend unending grace and hope to yourself. In this journey of health, remember that this is a steady race and not a sprint. Enjoy feeling your body move and experience health! Enjoy the journey.

> Just because we are not where we want to be in this moment does not mean that we don't have the ability to ever get to that place.

Body

Just because we are not where we want to be in this moment does not mean that we don't have the ability to ever get to that place. In your journal, I want you to write a letter of encouragement to yourself. It doesn't have to be long, but really allow yourself to be kind. What would you say to a friend who was on this same journey? Offer those same sweet words to yourself.

Soul

It's important to allow ourselves to receive grace when we are on this journey. There will always be mistakes made or lessons learned, but no moment that is learned from is ever wasted!

Spirit

Father, I thank You for the gift of grace. Please reveal to me any areas in my life where I am not giving myself grace and therefore robbing myself of the joy of the journey.

Week Six

ONE BITE OF SHAME

Go then, eat your bread in happiness and
drink your wine with a cheerful heart; for
God has already approved your works.
—ECCLESIASTES 9:7 NASB

Oftentimes, many emotions, memories, and internal beliefs come to mind when food is the subject at hand. Maybe food has been a lifelong struggle for you and you live in limbo between one fad diet after another. Maybe food brings feelings of guilt and the fear of weight gain or loss of control comes to mind. Or maybe you were raised in a family that celebrates food and used it to commemorate special events and life victories. No matter where you fall on the spectrum, one thing is the same— we all need food.

Have you ever stopped to wonder why food plays such a vital part in our emotional lives? How can something that doesn't have breath or words have the ability to make or break a person's day?

In Genesis, God placed Adam and Eve in the Garden of Eden. He gave them very specific instructions—eat anything you want except for the fruit from the tree in the middle of the garden. Satan was aware of these guidelines when he approached Eve one day.

> *"Did God really tell you not to eat fruit from any tree in the garden?"*
>
> *"We may eat the fruit of any tree in the garden," the woman answered, "except the tree in the middle of it. God told us not to eat the fruit of that tree or even touch it; if we do, we will die."*
>
> *The snake replied, "That's not true; you will not die. God said that because he knows that when you eat it, you will be like God and know what is good and what is bad"* (Genesis 3:1–5 GNT).

We all know what happened next. Eve gave in to the temptation of the devil and she ate the forbidden fruit. From that very moment, shame and guilt became associated with food. The curse of Eve has been carried through from generation to generation, and we still find ourselves in a battle with associating food with shame!

I invite you to allow yourself to release all shame that comes with food. Food was meant to bring life and to sustain us! Food was God's idea in the first place!

Food was meant to bring life and to sustain us! Food was God's idea in the first place!

Body

When we shift our mindset from shame to freedom, we actually are giving ourselves permission to enjoy food again! Today, I encourage you to give yourself permission to eat good, clean, and healthy foods. Before each meal, take a moment to thank God for the freedom in food that He has provided.

Soul

We were never created to live in shame! The curse of shame was brought upon us when Adam and Eve first sinned, but Christ has set us free from all sin and we now can live in freedom and victory!

Spirit

Father, I thank You that I no longer have to live in bondage toward food. I thank You that You have set me free and that I can now enjoy total freedom in You.

HONORING OUR BODIES WITH FOOD

For He has satisfied the thirsty soul, and the
hungry soul He has filled with what is good.
—PSALM 107:9 NASB

As we learned yesterday, food was God's idea and it was meant to bring us life and not shame! Our bodies were designed to crave and receive nutrients from the food that God has provided for us.

Our bodies were designed to feel good, full of life and energy. However, many of us feel just the opposite. Tired, lethargic, irritable, and unable to make it through the afternoon without a sugary treat or a cup of coffee. What we don't realize is that doing that only feeds into the cycle of food addiction and dependency in an unhealthy way.

Part of being a good steward of our body is learning how to honor our body with food. First Corinthians 10:31 says, "So whether you eat or drink, or whatever you do, do it all for the glory of God" (NLT). This verse shows us that God cares about what we eat and what we drink, and when we honor our bodies we honor the Lord!

A good way to help shift your mindset from "having" to eat healthy to "getting" to eat healthy is to think about the way your body will feel. After you eat a donut, do you feel energized or do you feel lethargic? After you eat fresh fruit or veggies, do you feel guilt-ridden or do you feel fueled and energized? We often associate food with weight loss or calories, but the key is to shift our mindset to focus on how we will *feel* when we choose to eat certain foods. This in itself is also a form of self-love because when we make a decision that is going to make us feel good, we are saying that we care about our bodies and our emotional health.

> The key is to shift our mindset to focus on how we will feel when we choose to eat certain foods.

Body

Today, I encourage you to be intentional about honoring your body. Take a moment to connect with it and feel what it needs to be successful today. Before you eat, think about whether your choices are going to honor or dishonor your body.

Soul

Our bodies were designed to be honored. Part of honoring God is learning how to honor our bodies. When we become intentional about treating our bodies well, our bodies will respond positively.

Spirit

Father, thank You for the gift of honor. I ask as I learn to honor You better that I also learn how to honor myself and my body. Please give me wisdom when making health and wellness choices today and give me the supernatural strength needed to honor You in every decision I make.

FULFILLMENT IN GOD

But for those who honor the Lord, his love lasts
forever, and his goodness endures for all generations.
—PSALM 103:17 GNT

We've all been there. The kids are acting crazy, the dishes are overflowing, the dog needs a bath, we were late for work again, and you and your spouse can't seem to agree on a single thing. We find ourselves overwhelmed, frustrated, and feeling unfulfilled. We may have all the good intentions in the world to make healthy choices, but all of that goes out the window and we find ourselves scrounging through our kitchen for something that will put our minds at ease. Ice cream, potato chips, stale cookies, anything that will help us avoid what's really going on inside of our hearts.

In the world we live in today, it is easy to go searching for a quick fix when we feel discomfort in our lives. It probably comes as no surprise to you that food addiction is actually one of the top addictions in America right now.[1] I could go into the science behind it and explain how the usage of GMOs and additives in our food play a part in this addiction, but I want to talk about the root of all addiction: the lack of fulfillment.

We were created to have needs. We all need love, attention, and relationships. Yes, some of those needs are meant to be met by friends and family. It is important for us to have healthy relationships in our lives. However, we will never find true fulfillment apart from God. Oftentimes, when we begin to feel disconnected from God or our own hearts, that causes us to feel discomfort. It is mere human nature to try to not feel uncomfortable, so we quickly scramble to try to feel comfortable again. This is not meant to be a bad thing as long as we are running to God for comfort instead of a temporary fix, such as food.

If you have found yourself struggling with food addiction or just simple emotional eating, I invite you to invite God in your struggle. In that moment when you want nothing more than to be hidden in the bathroom with a pint of ice cream, instead of giving in to your desires, turn your attention toward God and invite Him to come and meet you in your discomfort.

Invite Him to come and meet
you in your discomfort.

Body

Many of us may have unhealthy coping skills that we tend to run to when life gets hard. A key to breaking those addictions is finding a new and healthy coping skill. In your journal, make a list of at least ten activities that you can do when you feel the urge to turn to food or another substance for comfort. Often, I encourage people to keep your list with you so you can refer to it if you are out and about and need some extra support.

Soul

We were created to have needs, to have a comforter. However, if our source of comfort is found outside of God, we often are walking a dangerous path. It is important that we learn to run to God for refuge in the good times and bad.

Spirit

Father, I thank You that You are a source of strength for me. Thank You that I can turn to You for comfort and refuge at any time. I lay before You any unhealthy thought patterns or addictions that may get in the way of our relationship, and I ask that You give me the comfort I need in times of trouble.

Note

1. Jane Velez-Mitchell, "Top 5 Addictions in the U.S.," Addict Nation, accessed June 28, 2016, http://addictnation.org/top-5-addictions-in-the-u-s.

PRACTICING SELF-CONTROL

No temptation has overtaken you that is not common to man. God is faithful, and he will not let you be tempted beyond your ability, but with the temptation he will also provide the way of escape, that you may be able to endure it.
—1 CORINTHIANS 10:13 ESV

Growing up in church, I was often exposed to hearing about the fruits of the Spirit. Many Sunday school classes had felt boards with pictures of fruit, each representing different fruits of the spirit.

But the fruit of the Spirit is love, joy, peace, forbearance, kindness, goodness, faithfulness, gentleness and self-control (Galatians 5:22-23 NIV).

We know that as Christians we are to be people who show love, display joy, and bring peace to hard situations. However, one of the fruits of the Spirit often gets overlooked—self-control. Maybe you are someone who prides yourself on having a good sense of self-control, or maybe you are someone who struggles in this area. No matter where you are on the spectrum, the truth is that we all could afford to grow in this area.

There was a time in my life when I didn't have a very good grasp on self-control when it came to food. I was a sugar addict, and there were days I would eat an entire pound of chocolate in one day! My lack of self-control would come back to haunt me the next day when I would wake up feeling groggy and sick from all the sugar that I had consumed. When you're not feeling well, it's easy to take it out on your family or your spouse, which then causes them to feel unvalued. Lack of self-control can cause a vicious cycle in our lives and affect those around us.

When I began this journey toward health, I quickly learned that practicing self-control was going to be a huge aspect of this journey. My ability to control my earthly desires for sugar, carbs, and diet soda was going to either make or break this journey for me. In these moments, I had to quiet my heart and focus on my "Why." My "Why" is what gave me the ability to utilize self-control and say "no" to temptations and "yes" to health and wholeness.

We weren't created to feel powerless
and weak! The Spirit lives within us and
a fruit of the Spirit is self-control!

Body

What areas in your life could you use more self-control in? Take a moment to think about those areas and how having a lack of self-control negatively affects aspects of your life. Now imagine the ways practicing self-control could help positively affect your life. In your journal, write a short paragraph of how your life could look different in a month, a year, and five years from now if you focused on stewarding self-control. This will be a great reminder tool for those moments when you feel like giving up and throwing self-control out the window.

Soul

We weren't created to feel powerless and weak! The Bible says that the Spirit lives within us and a fruit of the Spirit is self-control! Learning how to manage our earthly desires will help bring us into a great part of our destiny.

Spirit

Father, thank You for the gift of self-control! I thank You You for giving me the power and ability to manage my cravings and desires. I ask that my desires will align with Your desires for me and that together we can move forward into greater blessings and increase as I learn to manage self-control in my life.

THE CYCLE OF COMPARISON

A heart at peace gives life to the
body, but envy rots the bones.
—PROVERBS 14:30 NIV

It seems like you can't go anywhere these days without hearing about the latest and greatest diet that promises a smaller waist and a happier, more fulfilled life. Vegan, paleo, vegetarian, Atkins, and south beach all sing their own praises and try to lure you in!

The truth is that there is no one-size-fits-all when it comes to eating, and it is easy to fall into the comparison trap. I have many friends who practice all different styles of eating. For me, if I tried to be like my friends who are vegan or vegetarian, I would fail miserably because my body needs meat to run efficiently. If I wasn't careful, I could then allow shame and comparison creep in, which could make me feel like a failure simply because my body was not designed the same way theirs was. Do you see how this could be a dangerous trap?

On the flip side, many of us may have friends who can stay perfectly slim while eating anything and everything that they want. That can also be a dangerous comparison trap, and we can find ourselves becoming bitter toward them or feeling shame toward ourselves. We have to remember that even though we may all be on the same journey, the roads we take look different at times.

Galatians 6:4-5 tells us, "Each of you must examine your own actions. Then you can be proud of your own accomplishments without comparing yourself to others. Assume your own responsibility" (GW). Wow! The freedom to examine our own actions gives us the freedom from having to compare our shortcomings with others!

> Even though we may all be on the same journey, the roads we take look different at times.

Body

Today, I want you to be intentional about paying attention to your thoughts. When you catch yourself comparing yourself or your progress with another person, I want you to stop and do two things. One, acknowledge what you love about the person you're comparing yourself to, as well as, acknowledge something that you love about yourself. For example, if you see someone with great hair and toned legs, you can say to yourself, "She looks amazing and I am happy for her. Maybe my legs aren't as toned as hers, but I work hard every day and I'm consistent with my workouts!" This practice not only helps take any root of jealousy away, but it also honors who both of you are.

Soul

Theodore Roosevelt said it best when he said, "Comparison is the thief of joy." Don't allow comparison to rob you of your journey and your potential.

Spirit

Father, I thank You for this journey toward wellness that I am on. Thank You that I can trust You to be my guide and to lead me where I need to go. Please help me protect my heart from comparison and help me remember how far You have already taken me.

Week Seven

THE ART OF LOVING OURSELVES

To acquire wisdom is to love yourself; people
who cherish understanding will prosper.
—PROVERBS 19:8 NLT

Have you ever spent time watching a young child as they go about life? Their curiosity and excitement is contagious as they explore the simple aspects of day-to-day life. They belly laugh when they find something funny and they cry when they feel hurt. They ask questions when they don't understand, without any fear of looking silly to others. When they catch themselves in a mirror, many times they will stop and smile at themselves, pose, and blow kisses. They like what they see and they aren't ashamed!

It makes you wonder, at what point did we lose that excitement and love for ourselves? Every person's story is different. Maybe it was a teacher who unknowingly hurt our feelings, or a parent who embarrassed us, or our peers. It doesn't help that we live in a society that teaches us that we are never good enough because there is always something that needs to be fixed. No matter what your story is, I have good news for you. You can begin to rewrite your story today.

Falling in love with yourself is not something that is done overnight. Many people want to just say one affirmation or kind thing about themselves and expect to wake up the next morning feeling completely different. Falling in love with yourself is often the same process as falling in love with another person. It takes time. Designated time is set aside to spend with that person, questions are asked, quirks are put on display, and traits are discovered. Over time, the person who was once a stranger suddenly becomes a part of who you are and you can't remember what life was like before you knew them. The same process holds true when we begin to fall in love with ourselves. At first, it may feel uncomfortable and awkward, but as you dig deeper and deeper into who you are, you will find that you will never want to live disconnected from yourself again.

> Falling in love with yourself is often
> the same process as falling in love
> with another person. It takes time.

Body

Today, I want you to take the time to get to know yourself. Write a letter to yourself as if you were introducing yourself to someone new. Tell them about your dreams, your quirks, and your favorite childhood memories. This will help you reconnect with who are and begin the process of learning to fall in love with who God created you to be.

Soul

As children, loving ourselves came easy because we didn't know any different. However, life has a way of making us believe lies. The good news is that we have the power to change those beliefs! It's never too late to fall in love with yourself and with life again!

Spirit

Father, I thank You for loving me unconditionally throughout my life. I ask that You now show me how to love myself in the same way. Today, I let go of any unhealthy beliefs and thought patterns that I've had about myself and I ask that You replace them with the truth. Help me see me through Your eyes.

BEAUTY IN CHRIST

You are altogether beautiful, my
darling, beautiful in every way.
—SONG OF SOLOMON 4:7 NLT

I have a friend who struggled with eating disorders most of her life, beginning as a young pre-teen. Her teenage years were filled with struggling with food obsession and a strong desire to lose weight. Eventually, her obsession turned into bulimia. After over a decade of battling with this disease and being at war with her body, she finally reached a point where she was willing to do anything to be free. She went before the Lord and asked for His guidance.

As she continued on her journey toward health and recovery, she began asking the Lord to show her how He saw her. You see, the Lord doesn't look at us and see our flaws, like we do. He looks at us and He sees Himself because He made us in His image. Over time, she began to see herself through His eyes and His beauty began to radiate within her.

In Song of Solomon 4:7, Solomon says to his bride, "You are altogether beautiful, my darling; there is no flaw in you" (NIV). I invite you to see that the Lord is saying the same to you. You are altogether beautiful. Considering that you were made in the image of God, how could you not be? In those moments when God so tenderly whispers the truth about you, we all have a choice to make. We can choose to believe it and allow the truth of His words to soak upon us, or we can choose to believe that He is lying and deny His love. I know that, for myself, I never want to belittle anything that the Lord says, so I choose to believe that He finds me beautiful.

I encourage you to really open your heart to receiving the truth from God today and every day. If you find that you have a hard time believing that you are beautiful, spend some time looking to Christ and asking Him what He has to say about you. I have a feeling that you will never be the same if you do.

> You are altogether beautiful. Considering that you were made in the image of God, how could you not be?

Body

Sometimes we can be so blinded by lies we believe about ourselves that we have hardly any idea where to begin searching for the truth. Today, I want you to ask a close friend or family member to tell you three things that they love about you. Write down what they say in a journal so you can reference back to it when you have a hard day. Really allow yourself to step into the truth of what they are saying.

Soul

We have been called *beautiful one* by God Himself! At the end of the day, His opinion is the only one that matters. Allow yourself to walk in His words and accept them as the truth of who you are. You are beautiful.

Spirit

Father, I thank You that You have seen me and You have called me beautiful. I repent for believing the lie that I am not beautiful or worthy of Your love and affection. Right now, I invite You to reveal to me just how beautiful I am and help me have the heart to receive it.

BREAKING SELF-SABOTAGE

It is for freedom that Christ has set us free.
Stand firm, then, and do not let yourselves
be burdened again by a yoke of slavery.
—GALATIANS 5:1 NIV

Self-sabotage is, sadly, a common struggle that runs rampant in our society. "Behavior is said to be self-sabotaging when it creates problems and interferes with long-standing goals."[1] I think we can all agree that at one point or another we have come face to face with the temptation of self-sabotage!

The apostle Paul even addressed the issue in Romans 7:15 when he said, "I don't really understand myself, for I want to do what is right, but I don't do it. Instead, I do what I hate" (NLT). You see, when Adam and Eve first sinned in the garden that in itself was a form of self-sabotage, which then set the desire to destroy our own flesh into motion. Adam and

Eve were tempted because Satan made them believe that they weren't "good enough" as they were. He intrigued them by telling them that they could be better, like God even, if they would just eat from the tree that they were instructed not to!

Self-sabotage stems from the belief that we are not good enough just as we are. When it comes to the journey of health, we often know before skipping our workout or eating more than our fair share of cake that it will only lead us to feeling sick. Yet we still make the decision to do it anyway, only to feel bad about ourselves in the end. It's like what Paul talked about in Romans—we do what we don't want to do, which brings us hurt in the end. This in itself is not an act of self-love but of self-sabotage.

To break the cycle of self-sabotage, we must let go of the belief that we aren't good enough or deserving of victory. In fact, we were designed for freedom and victory in Christ! When you face the temptation to give up, stand firm on the belief that you were created to be victorious.

> To break the cycle of self-sabotage, we must let go of the belief that we aren't good enough or deserving of victory. In fact, we were designed for freedom and victory in Christ!

Body

Today, I want you to repeat to yourself at least three times, "I deserve victory." Write it on a piece of paper or a notecard to carry around with you or even set a reminder in your phone and schedule it to alert you during the day. This will help align your mind with the truth as you go about your day.

Soul

Self-sabotage can be a tricky battle to fight because we don't always realize that we are doing it. However, when we become more aware of our thoughts and our patterns, we can stop going down its destructive path and begin living from a place of victory instead of defeat!

Spirit

Father, I thank You for a new day and a new chance to start again. Please help me become more aware of the destructive patterns that I may have created in my life and give me the supernatural tools I need to say goodbye to self-sabotage and hello to freedom in Christ.

Note

1. "Self-Sabotage," Psychology Today, accessed June 29, 2016, https://www.psychologytoday.com/basics/self-sabotage.

ACCEPTING YOUR BODY

So shall the king greatly desire thy beauty:
for he is thy Lord; and worship thou him.
—PSALM 45:11 KJV

If you are like me, you have found yourself standing in line at the grocery store face to face with a line of magazines that are filled with new diets, workout tricks, and a guaranteed sense of security if you just hand over the $5 and buy the magazine! It's easy to get sucked in, especially when we live in a culture where perfection is valued above anything else.

I believe that the trap that many people fall into is believing the lie that they will learn to love themselves once they lose a certain amount of weight or once they fit back into their jeans from high school. However, nothing could be further from the truth. The truth is, we need to be willing to love our bodies and ourselves and that includes accepting our flaws.

I know a lady who travels and speaks on the power of beauty. She struggled for years with not accepting herself and wishing she could change her body. When she travels, she brings mirrors and has the women in her group stand in front of them and speak to each part of their body, especially the parts that they wish they could change. They speak to their thighs and repent for the hateful comments that they have spoken over them and thank them for giving them the ability to sit and walk. They speak to their stomach and ask forgiveness for being so harsh and judgmental toward it and thank it for giving them the ability to enjoy foods. Many women experience great breakthrough in these sessions because not only does it help them break off agreement with the self-hate, but also it allows them to see their body for the powerful tool that it is!

I believe that many of us can afford to learn to fall in love with our bodies again. The truth is, maybe your body isn't at your goal weight yet or maybe your stomach hangs over your jeans more than you would like, but it is still your body and it fights every day to help keep you alive and allow you to experience the fullness of life. Let's stop the battle against our bodies and be brave enough to become friends and walk in the journey hand in hand with ourselves.

It is your body and it fights every day
to help keep you alive and allow you
to experience the fullness of life.

Body

Today, I want you to take a few moments and stand in front of the mirror and repent to your body for the negative words you have spoken over it. Then, declare at least five positive affirmations over yourself. Be intentional while doing this and really embrace the positive words that you are speaking over yourself. Remember, your words have power!

Soul

The love we have for ourselves should not be conditional. The key to lasting breakthrough is learning to love ourselves as we are in this very moment.

Spirit

Father, I thank You for Your unconditional love. I repent for believing the lie that I am not worthy of love just as I am. I ask that today will be the day I begin to love myself just as I am in this moment. Please help guide me and show me the things that You have created me to be that make me unique.

OUT OF HIDING

And we all, who with unveiled faces contemplate
the Lord's glory, are being transformed into
his image with ever-increasing glory, which
comes from the Lord, who is the Spirit.
—2 CORINTHIANS 3:18 NIV

We've all done it. We make a mistake. We feel ashamed for our actions. We feel embarrassed for the choices that we've made, and the safest thing to do is hide. We hide from our friends, our family, and even from God. Seclusion is only an illusion that allows us to believe that if we hide, we will stay safe. The only problem is that living in hiding is a dangerous way of life because it prevents those who love us from being able to help us.

It's much like when Adam and Eve hid from the Lord after they sinned. They became ashamed of themselves because they realized that they were naked. It wasn't the human body that ashamed them, it was the feeling of being exposed and seen for what they truly were. Instead of running to the Father, they ran and hid and tried to cover up their bodies in the hope that God wouldn't see them. We often do the same thing. When we make a mistake, the last thing we want is for God or our loved ones to see us. We don't want them to see us in our vulnerability because let's face it—vulnerability is scary. It's giving someone permission to see us outside of our strengths. However, the reward for allowing ourselves to be seen in those moments is often so much greater than the cost of hiding. It's in those moments that we can truly receive and feel love and acceptance. Those two things often bring healing to the wounded parts of our hearts.

If you continue to read the story of Adam and Eve, you will see that even after they sinned, God went looking for them. God is all-knowing. So we know that He was already well aware of what they had done, but that didn't stop Him from wanting to be with them. The same is true for us. We may feel shame for allowing our bodies to get to the weight we are or for snapping at our children or for running to food for comfort, but the truth is that even in those moments God still wants to be with us.

I encourage you to allow yourself to come out of hiding today. Make a commitment to yourself to allow yourself to be seen even in those moments when you want to hide.

The reward for allowing ourselves to be seen in those moments of vulnerability is often so much greater than the cost of hiding. It's in those moments that we can truly receive and feel love and acceptance.

Body

Give yourself permission to be vulnerable when you've made a mistake. Enlist a friend and share with them that you are on a journey of coming out of hiding and ask them to hold you accountable for not hiding anymore. You will find that there is so much more freedom in being honest in your mistakes!

Soul

Living in shame is just another way that the enemy tries to keep us secluded from community. When we allow ourselves to be vulnerable, it can be scary, but it also helps make us free.

Spirit

Father, I thank You for paying the ultimate price so that I no longer have to live in shame. I break all agreements that I have made with shame, known and unknown, and I declare that today is the day of change and breakthrough. I ask for a spirit of courage and bravery as I walk this new journey of freedom.

Week Eight

MAKING TIME FOR GOD

I say to the Lord, "You are my Lord; apart
from you I have no good thing."
—PSALM 16:2 NIV

My husband and I have been blessed to be able to spend a
lot of our time traveling and ministering at various churches all
over the world. While it can be exciting and ever-changing, it
can also become draining if we are not careful to be stewarding
our relationship with God. We make our relationship with God
a priority because, apart from Him, everything we do would be
worthless.

Our bodies are just a temporary means that carry us
through this life until we join the Father in the next. While it
is important to be taking care of our bodies while we are here,
we must be careful to not forsake taking care of our spirits.

Our spirits are the only things that we will be able to take from this earth to heaven.

As Christians, some of us may find ourselves jumping from one church function to the next. An easy trap to fall into is allowing ourselves to only spend time with God in a church service or meeting and forgetting to take personal one-on-one time with Him. Personally, I can feel a shift in my overall being if I go more than two to three days without spending time with Jesus. Oftentimes, if we are not making the time for God it is easy to become irritable, stressed, overwhelmed, or even depressed. That's because, just like our bodies were created to be fed actual food, our spirits were created to be fed from the Presence and Word of God! When we starve our spirit of its food, we become starved and are unable to function at our highest potential.

Jesus Himself understood the importance of making time for the Father. Luke 5:16 says, "Jesus often withdrew to lonely places and prayed" (NIV). He had such a value for His Father and time to be alone with Him that Jesus was not afraid to withdraw from the crowds that had gathered to see Him.

I believe that there is an intimacy that develops with God when we take the time out of our busy days to just spend time with Him. Sure, life can be stressful, busy, and demanding, but if we spend all our time trying to balance our life apart from God, what good is it all anyway? I encourage you to set aside even five minutes a day to just spend time with the Father. I can promise you that you have nothing to lose and everything to gain when you do.

When we starve our spirit of its food,
we become starved and are unable to
function at our highest potential.

Body

Take time to connect one on one with God. This can look like taking a walk while listening to worship music or praying, reading your Bible, or journaling. However you feel closest to God, take time to connect with Him.

Soul

Our relationship with God is the most important relationship we are going to have in our lives. Making the time to steward our relationship is the key to spirit health.

Spirit

Father, I thank You for giving me unlimited access to You. Help me to not take our relationship for granted but make daily time to spend with You so that we grow deeper and deeper in connection with each other.

THE HEART OF THE FATHER

Then you will call on me and come and
pray to me, and I will listen to you.
—JEREMIAH 29:12 NIV

My husband, Bill, and I have been married for over 40 years. We have had a wonderful marriage for many reasons, one being that we know how to communicate with one another. Imagine if throughout the 40-plus years we have been married that I never asked Bill a single question or gave him time to communicate his heart to me. On paper, we would still be married, but it probably wouldn't be a successful or even enjoyable marriage. I wouldn't actually know my husband. I wouldn't know his heart, his desires, or his dreams. I would only know the idea that I had of who he was. The same is true with the Lord.

Many Christians sadly go throughout their lives never actually getting to know the Lord. They know the concept of Him and they may even know what the Bible says about Him, but they don't actually *know* Him. They spend their relationship with Him doing all the talking and never allowing God to reveal Himself to them. If you find that you can relate to that, I have great news. God wants you to get to know Him!

Jeremiah 33:3 says, "Call to me and I will answer you, and will tell you great and hidden things that you have not known" (ESV). I love this verse because it tells us not only that God wants us to call upon Him, but He wants to entrust us with the secrets of His heart!

One of my favorite ways to connect with God is through soaking. Soaking is simply quieting the mind and the body and focusing all of your attention on the Lord. Often I will lay still with my eyes closed and play worship music. Sometimes I may have something weighing heavily on my heart, and sometimes my only goal is to just adore the Lord. When I do this, I open my mind and my spirit and give the Lord permission to reveal to me whatever is on His heart to show me. I've had many beautiful encounters with the Lord when I do this and I always leave feeling refreshed and connected.

God wants to share His heart with us. What a treasure to be given! I encourage you to not take advantage of such a gift and to pursue the heart of the One who loves you.

God wants you to get to know Him!
Not only does God want us to call
upon Him, but He wants to entrust
us with the secrets of His heart!

Body

My goal for you today is take one of your favorite worship songs and to soak throughout the entire song. Invite God to share with you what is on His heart and be open to receiving it. When you are done, I encourage you to take the time to journal what He showed you.

Soul

We were created to be in relationship with the Father. He longs to share His heart with us even more than we long to hear it!

Spirit

God, I thank You for the gift of Your heart. I ask that I never forsake the secret things of You. Give me a heart to know You more and ears to hear You in all circumstances!

CHRIST OUR ANCHOR

This hope is a strong and trustworthy
anchor for our souls. It leads us through
the curtain into God's inner sanctuary.
—HEBREWS 6:19 NLT

If you grew up in the church, you are most likely familiar with the hymn, "It Is Well." It is a song that has brought great peace and comfort to many in seasons of loss and defeat; however, many are not familiar with the heart-wrenching story behind why the song was penned.

Horatio G. Spafford was a successful lawyer from Chicago who lost most of his wealth and real estate investments in 1871 in the Great Chicago Fire just after the death of his son. In an effort to bring peace and healing to his wife and daughters, he scheduled a trip to Europe for his family. He sent his wife and daughters ahead and had planned to meet up with them. A few days after their departure, he received word that the boat carrying them had crashed leading to the loss of his daughters. Great grief and devastation overcame him and his wife as their world continued to crumble before their eyes. In a state of utter turmoil, he then got before the Lord where he penned the famous hymn that many of us have grown to love.

> *When peace, like a river, attendeth my way,*
> *When sorrows like sea billows roll;*
> *Whatever my lot, Thou hast taught me to say,*
> *It is well, it is well with my soul.*

While this story is tragic, there is a beauty in it. The beauty is that in the midst of incomprehensible pain and turmoil, he found Christ to be his anchor. Life is hard. While I believe in always seeking the joy in life, I am not blind to the fact that there is great sadness to be experienced in life. Divorce; the death of a friend, loved one, or child; bankruptcy; depression; and anxiety all have a way of bringing us to a place no one wants to experience. While pain is inevitable, Christ is always dependable.

> *So God has given both his promise and his oath. These two things are unchangeable because it is impossible for God to lie. Therefore, we who have fled to him for refuge can have great confidence as we hold to the hope that lies before us. This hope is a strong and trustworthy anchor for our souls. It leads us through the curtain into God's inner sanctuary* (Hebrews 6:18-19 NLT).

I love the fact that we have been given a "great confidence" in Christ. That great confidence doesn't mean that the pain of life hurts any less, but that we have a hope that we will be whole once again.

> While pain is inevitable, Christ
> is always dependable.

Body

In a journal, I want you to allow yourself to come face to face with your pain. Write everything that comes to your mind and don't hold back. Acknowledging our pain is a form of honoring our heart. When you are done, lay it before God and ask Him to show you His heart in the midst of your pain. How does He feel? How does he want to comfort you? Journal His response.

Soul

The trials of life can often feel overwhelming and defeating, but we have been given a hope and confidence in Christ our anchor!

Spirit

Father, I thank You for the gift of Christ. I thank You that even in the midst of great pain and tragedy that I will always have a confidence that comes through You. I ask for renewed hope and vision for my own life.

PRAYING THE SCRIPTURES

Pray then like this: "Our Father in heaven, hallowed
be your name. Your kingdom come, your will
be done, on earth as it is in heaven. Give us this
day our daily bread, and forgive us our debts, as
we also have forgiven our debtors. And lead us
not into temptation, but deliver us from evil."
—MATTHEW 6:9–13 ESV

The Word of God is one of the greatest gifts that we have been given. In it, we can see over and over the faithfulness and the goodness of God being displayed since the beginning of time. We see great men and women of faith on their journeys and can be encouraged by their strength while also learning from their shortcomings.

Hebrews 4:12 says, "For the word of God is living and active, sharper than any two-edged sword, piercing to the division of soul and of spirit, of joints and of marrow, and discerning the thoughts and intentions of the heart" (ESV). The Bible is living and active! Every time we take the time to read and spend time in the Word, our spirits are being fed while being made alive.

My good friends Wesley and Stacey Campbell have a beautiful message about taking the Bible and actually praying and declaring it over our lives. For years, they took verses out of the Bible and would pray them over their own lives as well as their families. They began to see great breakthrough in their lives as they allowed the power of the Word of God to take seed in their prayer lives.

Another example of using the power of the Word can be found in Matthew 4 when Jesus was in the wilderness.

During that time the devil came and said to him, "If you are the Son of God, tell these stones to become loaves of bread." But Jesus told him, "No! The Scriptures say, 'People do not live by bread alone, but by every word that comes from the mouth of God.'" Then the devil took him to the holy city, Jerusalem, to the highest point of the Temple, and said, "If you are the Son of God, jump off! For the Scriptures say, 'He will order his angels to protect you. And they will hold you up with their hands so you won't even hurt your foot on a stone.'" Jesus responded, "The Scriptures also say, 'You must not test the Lord your God.'" Next the devil took him to the peak of a very high mountain and showed him all the kingdoms of the world and their glory. "I will give it all to you," he said, "if you will kneel down and worship me." "Get out of here, Satan," Jesus told him. "For the Scriptures say, 'You must worship the Lord your God and serve only him.'" *Then the devil went away, and angels came and took care of Jesus* (Matthew 4:3–11 NLT).

Jesus used the Word of God to combat the enemy, and the enemy eventually gave up trying to tempt Him! What a powerful tool we have such access to! We can all learn from this story as we can see the power that the Scriptures carry.

> Jesus used the Word of God to combat the enemy, and the enemy eventually gave up trying to tempt Him!

Body

Ask the Holy Spirit to reveal two or three scriptures that He wants you to focus on. I encourage you to write them down and keep them in a place that you have easy access to. Throughout your day, pray those scriptures over your life and your family.

Soul

The Bible is the most powerful tool that we have been given as believers! It carries life, breakthrough, and truth that has the ability to make the enemy flee from us!

Spirit

Father, I thank You for the gift of Your Holy Word. I pray that as I read Your Scriptures my body, soul, and spirit will all be brought to life under its authority.

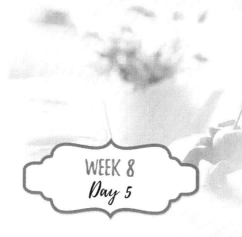

THE POWER OF WORSHIP

Let everything that has breath praise
the Lord. Praise the Lord.
—Psalm 150:6 NIV

One of the greatest men to have ever lived was best known for his worship. King David lived a great life of favor in the eyes of God. I love the story and the life of David because it shows us that even when we completely miss the mark and make mistakes, God is quick to restore and forgive.

I believe that worship plays an important part in the life of a Christian, and this can be seen in David's life. The Psalms are full of the words and music that David poured forth before the Lord whether in seasons of victory or defeat. Worship not only honors God, but it brings our beings into alignment with Him. It is the key to breakthrough in all areas of our lives. We know that David understood this because we see him worshiping before the Lord through every season in his life.

One of my favorite stories in the Bible is the story of King Jehoshaphat. When he had received word that an enemy nation was closing in to attack, instead of planning an attack in return he decided to send forth the musicians to worship.

> *After consulting the people, the king appointed singers to walk ahead of the army, singing to the Lord and praising him for his holy splendor. This is what they sang: "Give thanks to the Lord; his faithful love endures forever!" At the very moment they began to sing and give praise, the Lord caused the armies of Ammon, Moab, and Mount Seir to start fighting among themselves. The armies of Moab and Ammon turned against their allies from Mount Seir and killed every one of them. After they had destroyed the army of Seir, they began attacking each other. So when the army of Judah arrived at the lookout point in the wilderness, all they saw were dead bodies lying on the ground as far as they could see. Not a single one of the enemy had escaped* (2 Chronicles 20:21–24 NLT)

How many of us have faced a trial in our lives and have exhausted our energy trying to fight it on our own terms, only to be defeated? We can learn from both King David and King Jehoshaphat and change the way we go about fighting. We should worship! Whatever season you are in, whether a season of joy or of grief, I encourage you to never go a day without worship.

Worship not only honors God, but it brings our beings into alignment with Him. It is the key to breakthrough in all areas of our lives.

Body

Spent the next five to ten minutes in worship. Some like to worship through song, some like to dance, while others like to write out their praise to God. Whatever you like to do, set aside time to really worship.

Soul

Worship is the key to breakthrough! It brings our spirits in alignment with God's and allows us to experience His presence.

Spirit

Father, I thank You for creating me to worship You! As I worship, may Your presence would surround me. Reveal to me Your heart and give me an open heart to receive what You have for me!

ABOUT BENI JOHNSON

Beni Johnson is a bestselling author, pastor, and conference speaker. Together, she and her husband, Bill Johnson, are the Senior Overseers of Bethel Church in Redding, California. Beni has traveled all over the world bringing a message of joy, intercession, and now health in body, soul, and spirit. Beni is a mother to three children, along with their spouses, and the grandmother to nine grandchildren.

Healthy & Free

A JOURNEY TO WELLNESS FOR YOUR BODY, SOUL, AND SPIRIT

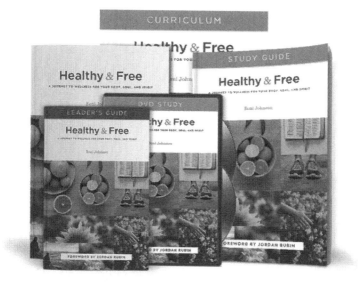

Experience Heaven's Health!

Beni Johnson received a life-changing revelation about how anyone can start walking in holistic health—including you! Jesus died for your spirit, soul, and body. This means you can experience His resurrection life in all three areas!

Christians should be the healthiest people on earth because they understand God has made their bodies His temple. Unfortunately, many people focus on one area of health while neglecting the others. This can lead to spiritual disconnection, bad eating habits, depression, poor rest, and lack of exercise.

In the *Healthy and Free* video curriculum, Beni personally teaches you how to:

- **Find your why:** Learn the motivating secret to pursuing a healthy lifestyle as your new normal.
- **Unlock the connection:** Discover the many ways your spirit, soul, and body are interconnected and how health in one area directly affects another.
- **Start simple:** Receive practical and easy-to-implement steps to begin walking in health right now.

The Great Physician desires you to walk in Heaven's health. Get aligned with God's divine design today and experience freedom—body, soul, and spirit!

INCLUDED IN THIS CURRICULUM:

8-Session DVD Study • Leader's Guide • Study Guide • *Healthy and Free* Book

YOUR HEALTHY & FREE LIFESTYLE IS JUST ONE DECISION AWAY...

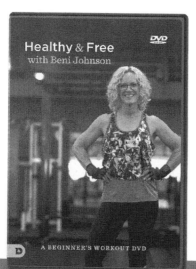

Healthy & Free
with Beni Johnson

DVD

A BEGINNER'S WORKOUT DVD

EXERCISE.

In this workout DVD, Beni Johnson gives you fun, easy-to-follow exercises that leave you without excuse.

She makes working out so easy and fun that no matter how busy your schedule is, you can still make one of the most important investments of all: a healthy lifestyle!

Beni gives you over two hours of exciting and enjoyable workouts that will show you...

- How to exercise anywhere... from the comfort of your own home to the scenic environment of a park
- How to comfortably and effectively use equipment in your home
- How to confidently use gym machines to maximize your workout impact and effectiveness

Once you begin the journey and start feeling the results in your body, you will make working out a regular part of your schedule that will set you on course for a lifetime of living healthy and free!

FREE E-BOOKS?
YES, PLEASE!

Get **FREE** and deeply discounted **Christian books** for your **e-reader** delivered to your inbox **every week!**

IT'S SIMPLE!

VISIT lovetoreadclub.com

SUBSCRIBE by entering your email address

RECEIVE free and discounted e-book offers and inspiring articles delivered to your inbox every week!

Unsubscribe at any time.

SUBSCRIBE NOW!

LOVE TO READ CLUB

visit **LOVETOREADCLUB.COM** ▶

Printed in Great Britain
by Amazon